Legal & Disclaimer

The information contained in this book is not designed to replace or take the place of any form of medicine or professional medical advice. The information in this book has been provided for educational and entertainment purposes only.

The information contained in this book has been compiled from sources deemed reliable, and it is accurate to the best of the Author's knowledge; however, the Author cannot guarantee its accuracy and validity and cannot be held liable for any errors or omissions. Changes are periodically made to this book. You must consult your doctor or get professional medical advice before using any of the suggested remedies, techniques, or information in this book.

Upon using the information contained in this book, you agree to hold harmless the Author from and against any damages, costs, and expenses, including any legal fees potentially resulting from the application of any of the information provided by this guide. This disclaimer applies to any damages or injury caused by the use and application, whether directly or indirectly, of any advice or information presented, whether for breach of contract, tort, negligence, personal injury, criminal intent, or under any other cause of action.

You agree to accept all risks of using the information presented inside this book. You need to consult a professional medical practitioner in order to ensure you are both able and healthy enough to participate in this program.

Table of Contents

INTRODUCTION

It is no surprise at all that our bodies slow down as we age. With each additional candle on the birthday cake, you probably will notice that your strength and stamina is a far cry from your youthful sports hero days, you are not as quick on your hands and feet as you used to be, you may also have become more susceptible to falling sick, and – perhaps most obvious of all – your waistline may have significantly expanded.

Vanity issues aside, weight gain in your 50s is not to be taken lightly. Being overweight is known to heighten a person's risk of heart disease, diabetes, cancer and many other chronic illnesses – risks which increase even more as you get older. Additionally, your joint health would suffer, thus compromising your mobility and overall quality of life. Can you imagine life in your golden years to be filled with frequent hospital visits, taking medication on clockwork, and missing out on holiday family jaunts because of your limited mobility? Well, here is the good news: you do not have to resign yourself to such a hopeless fate. Even if you have been living a sedentary lifestyle with poor dietary habits, it is never too late to put the brakes on the scale's rising number and regain control of your health. It is only too late if you allow it to be so!

This guide does not come with a promise of rapid weight loss either, because healthy and long-term weight loss cannot be realistically achieved with a few tips and tricks. It involves making gradual but lasting changes to a few key aspects of one's lifestyle.

What you are about to learn in the following chapters will not require you to spend a lot of money on health supplements, following some fad diet, or be subjected to extreme and potentially harmful weight loss measures. Everything outlined here are natural weight loss methods that takes into account the physiological changes of aging, and how you can work around them in ways that are beneficial to your own well-being.

You will learn why weight loss after 50 has to be approach differently, what are the best exercises to regain some of the vitality you took for granted during your youth, and the best dietary practices for prudent weight management without compromising your enjoyment of food. You will also learn about lifestyle habits that are sabotaging your weight loss efforts, and health red flags to watch out for. All these are scientific-based tried-and-true methods that – if followed through with diligence – can help you achieve your weight loss goals, and reap the multiple health benefits that come with it.

Aging is an inevitable process, but the outlook does not have to be bleak at all. With the right knowledge and sensible lifestyle choices, it is possible to look and feel your best inside out, and enjoy life to the fullest. All you have to do on your part is to take action and be in charge of your life once more.

CHAPTER 1

BE FIT AFTER 50

The big five-oh is an age milestone that brings about a lot of physiological changes – both visible and subtle – that significantly impacts one's general health and well-being. Aging is a fact of biology that slowly makes itself known in several visible ways. You may have noticed the number on the weighing scale is significantly higher than it were a decade or two ago. Plus, you no longer have the stamina, strength and agility to endure grueling workouts to shed the weight as you were used to in your heydays. However, that does not mean you have to let yourself go.

Staying in shape is not just about looking good or being able to outdo someone half your age; your overall quality of life is at stake here. There are unseen dire health consequences that come with the weight gain. Being overweight or obese increases your risk of conditions like high blood pressure, high cholesterol, osteoarthritis and sleep apnea – silent killers which can lead to more serious illnesses if left unchecked. This is especially a cause for concern in your 50s as your body's resistance to diseases is also on the decline.

With all things considered, it is an understatement to say that being fit after 50 is crucial. Sure, losing and maintaining the ideal weight in your golden years may not be as easy as it was in your 20s and 30s, but it is not a farfetched feat one might think. Before diving into another weight loss program, you need to first understand the changes the body goes through as we get older, how that affects our ability to lose weight and what we can do about it.

Metabolism and the Aging Process

Remember back in your 20s when binge eating pizza and get sloshed was the typical weekend ritual? You may have gained a few pounds over time, but when swimsuit season comes around in summer, you can just cut down on the partying and calories, then whipped yourself back into shape with extra time at the gym. Well, why can't you shed the weight as fast as you used to anymore? This has to do with your metabolism slowing down.

Metabolism is the rate at which the body converts calories from food into energy to be used as fuel for natural bodily functions and daily activities. The minimum amount of calories burned with bodily functions – such as breathing, digestion, keeping vital organs working etc. – is known as basal metabolic rate (BMR). Each person's BMR is different, and is directly affected by age, gender, weight, and physical activities. The higher one's BMR, the quicker calories get burned up rather than stored as fat. Generally, there are two factors that the BMR can be increased:

1. **Exercising** – Your BMR can stay raised after 30 minutes of moderate physical activity, and can stay increased for about 48 hours following intense exercise.

2. **Increased muscle mass** – Unlike fats, muscles are metabolic; they use more energy than fat cells, even

while resting or sleeping. The more muscle tissue one has, the more energy their body uses. Hence, people with more muscle mass tend to have higher BMR.

In theory, for weight loss to happen, one has to use up additional calories by maintaining an active lifestyle and following proper dietary habits that prevents accumulation of unused calories. However, it is hardly as straightforward because there are many factors than can affect your BMR, including aging.

The body normally starts aging after 30, where many physiological processes begin to decline, but the signs do not become obvious until the age of 50 onwards. On average, the metabolism slows down by 5-10% per decade after one turns 30. Here are some biological factors that decline with each passing birthday, thus contributing to lower metabolism:

- Number of cells in each organ drops
- Bone density decreases
- The amount of muscle mass decreases due to the decline in quantity and size of muscle fibers
- Strength peaked in the early to mid-30s, and then begin dropping by 8% per decade
- Cardiac output (the heart's ability to pump blood) and oxygen volume diminishes with each decade by roughly 5% each decade, resulting in decreased cardiovascular endurance
- Approximately 8-10cm of lower back and hip flexibility will be lost as we age; an accumulation of both longstanding lifestyle habits and loss of collagen (an important structural protein in connective tissue that holds the body together)

These are the factors accountable for the overall reduction of physical activity, which further contributes to slowing down one's metabolism.

Too Late to Lose Weight?

If you have been exercising regularly and eating healthy for most of your adult life, the effects of a declining metabolism may not have a big impact on your fitness well-being. In which case, keep up the good work! On the other hand, if you have been leading a sedentary lifestyle, with a diet that predominantly consists of fatty processed foods, sugary beverages and alcohol, it is never too late to reform your lifestyle.

Metabolism does take a downward slide with age, but it is possible to offset this effect with the appropriate eating and exercise plan, regardless of your age. In fact, to be fit after 50 not only keep you going by slowing down your body's gradual decline, it also offsets your risks of many deadly diseases. However, while weight loss at an older age is definitely achievable, it is not the same as trying to lose weight when you were younger. Because your body is not as formidable anymore, there are precautions to take before attempting a weight loss program.

Ideally, you want to see a doctor for a full health assessment, and have a discussion about your weight loss goals. You need to take into account your physical limitation, which could mean checking with your doctor if it is safe for you to partake in intensive exercises. If you have been diagnosed with a certain health condition and put on long-term medication, you also need to know what types of foods don't belong in your diet.

In the next three chapters, you will be guided about the best exercises, foods and lifestyle choices that can be adopted to help melt away the excess pounds. Whenever in doubt, consult a qualified healthcare professional. Just remember that you are never too old to be fit!

CHAPTER 2

AGE GRACEFULLY WITH EXERCISE

When it comes to losing weight, nothing can substitute a good exercise program. An active body burns more calories, store less excess fat, stay stronger and maintains greater mobility – it is as simple as that. Regular physical activity does a lot more than just making number on the scale drop; many age-related declines happening to the body can be offset by maintaining an active lifestyle.

To maximize your weight loss potential and ensure you benefit from improved mobility, you need to opt for an exercise program that addresses the three major areas of physical fitness, which are flexibility, strength and aerobic fitness. Let's examine how you can begin setting up a program for yourself that meets your weight loss and fitness needs.

Built the Habit and Aerobic Fitness

If you have never consistently followed a fitness plan before, it is not wise to dive straight into a formal workout program. Your body is not used to the shock and stress of exercising, which puts you at risk of injuring yourself. Plus, to wake up feeling tired and sore post-workout can be discouraging, making it tempting to quit. Instead of going into warrior mode and hit the gym following years of being inactive, you want to start small and gradually built up the stamina, strength and mobility to endure longer and more intense workouts.

Start by training yourself to get into the habit of allocating time for physical activity each day. The simplest way to do this is by taking a leisurely stroll around the block or at a nearby park. You can also walk on a treadmill; what matters is you get moving. In order to endure more intense exercises, you need to have a degree of aerobic fitness– also known as cardiovascular fitness – as a foundation. Walking is the safe and most accessible form of exercise that anyone, regardless of fitness level, can do to begin incorporating physical activity into their daily routine. Furthermore, walking is a form of aerobic exercise that gets your heart pumping. In addition, you are already burning some calories with walking.

To start off, choose a safe environment to walk where the air is fresh and there are no road hazards, and put on proper shoes that gives your feet comfortable cushioning when you walk. It would be best if you can get into a walking routine in the morning, shortly before or after a light breakfast. Doing something aerobic in the morning in beneficial in many ways; the morning air is fresher and you will feel more energized throughout the day. Moreover, a light exercise after getting out of bed and before packing on more calories with meals later actually forces the body to cash in on stored fat.

You don't need to be too hard on yourself; just start off with 5-15 minutes for 3-4 days a week. Gradually, work on building up to an hour by adding 5-10 minutes to your daily walks. IF you do this dedicatedly, you should feel your stamina improving and the walks become easier. Once you can manage walking for one hour, you can than make things more challenging by turning walking at a faster pace. You can also use ankle weights for added resistance, but don't strap weights on your wrist as it can be harmful to your shoulder.

After about 8-12 weeks, you may be ready to switch things up by cutting your walking time in half and use the remainder time for other exercises you enjoy. For people who cannot handle other workouts like dance, yoga or weights due to certain medical conditions, a regular routine of brisk to moderate-paced walking will work wonders for your heart health, and when coupled with a good diet, is enough to shed some pounds.

For optimal benefit or any aerobic workout, you want to be able to reach a heart rate of 120-150 beat per minute (bmp). This is known as the fat-burning zone that will crank up your metabolism temporarily for the next 30 minutes to 48 hours, depending on the intensity of your workout.

Yoga: The Mind-Body-Spirit Workout

Flexibility is an indicator of joint health and the key to good range of motion. It is safe to say there is no better form of workout for improving flexibility than yoga. Originating from India some thousands of years ago, yoga has now become one of the more popular fitness systems around the world. Yoga's appeal lies in the fact that it is an accessible and comprehensive workout for the mind, body and spirit, which can also act as a non-religious spiritual practice anyone can incorporate into their daily lives.

The practice of yoga comprises of deep meditation, breathing techniques, and a series of physical exercise where one transitions from various postures known as *Asana*. Each aspect of the practice is intended to benefit various aspects of one's mental and physical health. Yoga is especially beneficial for those over 50 because of its low-impact, non-competitive and therapeutic nature. With prolonged consistent practice, it is said that yoga can reverse many of the age-related deterioration in the body. The multitude of benefits to be had from yoga includes:

- Relieve stress, anxiety and depression
- Better mental focus and clarity of thought
- Improved mood and emotional stability
- Improved skin elasticity and radiance
- Detoxifies the body
- Hormonal and nervous system balance
- Improved flexibility and range of motion
- Improved spinal and joint health
- Improved strength and muscle tone
- Steady weight loss and maintenance
- Better standing posture and balance
- Higher metabolism
- Therapeutic for recovering and rehabilitation from injury
- Relieve chronic pain in the body
- Relieve migraines and headaches
- General lowered risk of various chronic illnesses
- More self-confidence

These claims were not exaggerated though; plenty of scientific research has been conducted in the western world since the 1970s has testified to yoga's effectiveness. After all, a system would not have stood the test of time if it is nothing more than a fad!

For those who have never tried yoga, it can be a challenge to get their feet wet into the practice. You may find the yoga postures to be intimidating, perhaps thinking you do not have the strength and flexibility to survive a class. Do not let all the bendy postures deter you! Sure, there are hundreds of yoga *asanas* to be learned, but the goal of practicing is not to be able to get into all of them. Yoga is a transformative workout that focuses on the inner journey. Postures are achieved through gradual practice, building up the strength, balance and flexibility at your own pace. In other words, your practice is meant to benefit you, and there is no competition of who can bend and twist themselves into complicated postures. Additionally, there is a huge sense of accomplishment and empowerment for pushing yourself beyond your comfort zone, and being able to pull off a posture you never thought was possible before.

Given yoga's extensive history, the practice had sprouted various branches of different traditions and styles. There are certain styles that are more suited to relaxation, some are more therapeutic, and then there are those which are very physically demanding. With so many styles, there are many yoga studios and even vacation retreats, offering courses to yogis of all ages and fitness levels.

Yoga can be your sole fitness practice, or you can incorporate it into your weight loss program to supplement other workouts. If you intend on beginning the practice, assuming that a doctor has given you the green light, follow these pointers:

- **Be clear of what you want to gain from yoga and choose the style that suits your need.** Take your time and do some research on the different yoga styles, their history and specific health benefits. Most yoga teachers practice hybrids of various styles, and ended up formulating their own. When you look for a yoga studio to join, ask if there have instructors whose style specializes in addressing your needs.

- **Study under a good teacher.** The instructor – known as a guru – which you choose to study can make all the difference. A competent guru can guide a beginner through the practice, provide modifications and alternatives to challenging postures, and teaches students how to properly safeguard themselves from injury when trying out an unfamiliar posture. A guru should under no circumstance exert their authority to pressure and force a student into attaining a posture! Yoga is not boot camp and that just defeats the whole purpose of practice.

- **Prepare yourself.** If you feel apprehensive about stepping into a yoga class with zero knowledge, why not teach yourself some beginner postures, so you would know what to expect? There are plenty of resources – books, home videos and websites – where you can pick up basic *asanas.*

- **Don't neglect the spiritual element.** Yoga has its roots in Hinduism and philosophy, although it is non-religious and does not interfere with an individual's faith. While it is no doubt a beneficial workout, a lot of modern schools tend to neglect its spiritual element. There are some studios that teach a more orthodox style where teachers would encourage students to incorporate the spiritual practice of yoga into their lives. If such is the case with the studio that you joined, be open to it. You will be surprise at the profound inner peace to be had from being more spiritual.

Strength Training is not just for the young and hip!

Building physical strength is necessary as you get older, not just to prevent further loss in muscle mass and metabolism decline, but also to maintain bone density. Greater physical strength comes from resistance training, and there are two main systems for that: weights and calisthenics – both when paired with a protein and calcium-rich diet, are effective in improving muscle mass and strengthen bones, even after age 50.

Weight training utilizes fitness equipments and machines for resistance, normally requiring you to train in a gym. Meanwhile, callisthenic workouts use the weight of your own body for resistance. Whichever workout you opt for depends on preference, and to a certain degree, your current state of health and level of fitness. For instance, if you suffer from shoulder and knee pain, pushups and squats may not be doable. If you have stiff joints, lifting heavy weights may be too strenuous and cause injury. A well-structured strength routine is often one which incorporates the best of both training methods.

However you choose to strength train, be sure your workout does not neglect all the major upper and lower body muscle groups, and also the core. You can also incorporate cardio/aerobic workout into your resistance training routine to benefit the heart and maximize calorie torching. Here are a few simple examples of strength exercises which you can start with at the comfort of your home, with minimal equipment. These workouts combined weight lifting and calisthenics, and only requires a pair of dumbbells and a pair of ankle weights:

Upper body (chest, back, shoulders, biceps and triceps)

Standing dumbbell curls (also known as bicep curls)

1. Stand with your feet shoulder-width apart.
2. Hold a dumbbell in each hand, and rotate your wrists so that palms and fingers face forward.
3. Inhale and bend both arms at the elbows, lifting the dumbbells up to shoulder height.
4. Exhale and lower both arms.
5. Repeat 10-20 times.

Seated (or standing) dumbbell shoulder presses

1. Sit on a chair with your back straight, knees shoulder-width apart, with feet flat on the floor and aligned with the knees. If you choose to stand, make sure feet are shoulder-width apart and back straight.
2. Hold a dumbbell in each hand and raise them to shoulder height, and rotate your wrists so that palms and fingers face forward. If done correctly, your elbows should be aligned with your shoulders, and your forearm pointing straight up at 90-degrees.
3. Take a deep inhale, and as you exhale, push the dumbbells upward until the touch at the top, over your head.
4. Pause for 2 seconds, and slowly lower the weights back down to starting position while inhaling.
5. Repeat 10-20 times.

Wall pushups

1. Stand arm's length away from a wall with your feet shoulder-width apart.
2. Place your palms flat on the wall and, keeping your body straight and your core engaged.
3. Inhale and lean towards the wall. Hold for a second before slowly pushing yourself back to starting position while exhaling.
4. Repeat 10-20 times.

* This is a super easy version of pushups. Gradually, increase the body's angle by pressing up from a sturdy table or bench, until you build up the strength to do pushups with hands on the floor. When you make a transition to doing real pushups, you can modify it with knees on the floor, until you become strong enough to do so from a full plank position.

Lower body (buttocks, quadriceps, hamstrings and calves)

Side-lying leg raises

1. Lie on your left side with your body in a straight line, knees together, head supported on your left forearm and hold your core tight.
2. Slowly lift your right leg as high as you can and pause.
3. Slowly lower your leg to starting position.
4. Repeat 10-20 time, and switch sides.
* Don't tense your neck; keep it relaxed.

Standing hip extension

1. Strap on ankle weights, and stand straight with your hands on the back of a sturdy chair or railing for support.
2. Raise your left leg behind you, keeping your toes pointed at the floor while trying to lift your leg to hip height, keeping your back straight and gaze straight ahead.
3. Slowly lower your leg and foot back down until your foot is almost, but not quite, touching the floor.
4. Repeat 10-20 times, and switch legs.

Wall sits

1. Stand with feet shoulder-width apart and at a step's distance away from the wall.
2. With your feet in the same position, gently lean back against the wall.
3. With the back of your head to your buttocks are flat against the wall, slowly slide down, activating you thighs and butt muscles. You can move your feet forward if needed, but make sure both sides are parallel, so you are not working one leg more than the other.
4. You want to arrive at a position where your knees are at 90-degrees, while your back is still pressed against the wall. If this is too difficult for you, lower down until your knees are at 45-degrees.
5. Hold for 30 seconds to 1 minute.
6. Push yourself off the wall into a standing position when you are done.

Core (abdominals, hips and lower back)

Bird dogs

1. Get on your hands and knees, align your wrists under your shoulders, and your knees under the hips. Brace your core.
2. With a deep inhale, simultaneously raise your right arm straight out in front of you and your left leg straight out behind you.
3. Hold for 3 seconds and then slowly lower and return to starting position.
4. Repeat 10-20 times, and switch sides.

Reverse crunches

1. Lie down flat on the floor, with legs straight, arms by your side with palms facing down on the floor, and bring your feet together.
2. Lift your feet off and bend your knees to 90-degrees.
3. Inhale, suck in the lower belly, and lift your buttocks off the floor slightly, pulling your knees close to your chest using the strength of your abdominals.
4. Pause, and return back to starting position. Do not lower your feet back to the floor until you are done.
5. Repeat 10-20 times.

Plank

1. Get into the pushup startup position, with your palms on the floor, legs straight, and abdominals tightened and activated.
2. Look straight down at the space between your palms; do not let your neck droop down and keep it activated.

3. Take deep inhales and exhales for a count of 10 breaths, or hold the position for 30 seconds. Gradually, work up to holding it for a minute.

Weight/resistance-bearing Cardio

Jogging in place

Jog in the same spot by lifting the knees until it aligns with the hips alternately vigorously swinging your arms in coordination for 30 seconds to 1 minute. This can be done as a pre-workout warm-up. Due to the high intensity and impact, do not do this exercise if you have bad knees.

Jumping jacks

1. Start by standing straight, with your feet together and hands by your side.
2. Take a deep inhale and jumping your feet a bit wider than shoulder-width apart, while raising your hands above your head and clapping them.
3. As soon as your hands clapped and your feet touch the ground, immediately jump back into starting position.
4. Repeat 10-20 times.

* This is an intense and explosive workout. Do not do jumping jacks if you have bad knees or joint pains.

Weekly Workout Template

For measurable results, you need to dedicate at least 3-4 days per week, for a total time of 150-200 minutes. That means each workout session should last a minimum of 50 minutes. Don't worry if you cannot manage that; remember that you can always start small and work your way up to exercising for 200 minutes per week. Even if you have been a couch potato most of your life and is just starting to get serious about fitness at 50, you can begin by giving 5-15 minutes to each session. What's important is that you are doing something to try shedding the pounds.

The following is a sample workout plan that covers the three important areas of fitness. Feel free to customize it to suit your personal fitness level and needs.

- 15-30 minutes brisk walking every other day
- 15 minutes of yoga for 2 days
- 4 strength exercises for 10 repetitions each for 2 days (on days when not doing yoga)

The more you stick to your plan, you will feel your workout gets easier and you are not exerting yourself much for each session. This is a sign that you are making progress! It means your strength, flexibility and stamina are improving. When you feel that is starting to happen, it means it's time to step things up. Increase the repetitions and durations of the exercises that you do or try more advanced exercises; find new ways to challenge yourself.

The 10 Commandments of being 50 and Fit

1. **Get moving.** You can maximize your calorie burning by taking up a physical activity you enjoy in addition to your workout program. How about signing up for a ballroom dancing class? Or join a local charity walk?

Or volunteer at an event that keeps you on your feet? You can also get into the habit of parking the car further and walk more, or take the stairs instead of the elevator.

2. **Go easy on the Joints.** Tired and painful joins can be a hindrance to your weight loss goals. If you suffer from joint problems, opt for activities that are light-impact, so as not to let the aches and pains put you off from exercising. Activities like water aerobics, swimming, walking, kayaking, cycling and yoga are gentle on the joints.

3. **Always switch things up.** Humans are creatures of habits, and so is every cell and fiber in our bodies. When you become accustomed to a certain type of exercise or routine, it eventually becomes less challenging. Have variety in your workout program. For example, don't do the same strength exercises in the same week, have a new yoga routine each session, and alternate between walking, cycling and dancing for your cardio needs. You don't want to get bored of exercising, because then it is easy to lose track of your weight loss goals.

4. **Do the things you enjoy.** Are your exercises boring you? Then opt for an alternative for your aerobic health, like dancing, Pilates, step aerobics, swimming or organize a weekend hiking trip for the family.

5. **Pace Yourself.** Remember that your primary goal is weight loss and maintenance, and you are not in competition with anyone. Even the top athletes will tell you that you can't return to the peak physicality as you once had in your prime. So, keep your health and well-being in mind above all else. The last thing you want is to collapse from over-exercising.

6. **Listen to your body.** It does not pay to overexert yourself! Remember, you are in competition with no one else but yourself. So, take it easy and slowly coach – not coax – yourself into fitness.

7. **Have a workout buddy.** Exercising and losing weight with another person is a wonderful way to kick boredom and stay motivated. So, talk to a friend or get your spouse involve in your workout goals, and ask them to join you. Likewise, you can make friends and exchange weight loss tips with folks from your fitness classes and gym.

8. **Make days for rest and recovery.** Your body needs time to rest and recover from the strain of exercising. So, take days off between working out to rest out the muscle sores.

9. **Be disciplined and make no excuses.** It's often tempting to not hit the gym when you feel tired and achy all over. You won't be seeing results if you keep slacking from your program! If you feel soreness or pain, either from working out or other health condition, make adjustments to your exercise program to accommodate your condition. You can always turn things down a notch or take an extra day rest, just as long as you are not straying too far from your weight loss goals.

10. **Have realistic expectations.** Weight loss cannot happen overnight. To prevent yourself from feeling discouraged and obsess over your weight, avoid the temptation of weighting yourself or taking body measurements too frequently. It is best to track your progress by doing a critical mirror assessment every 2-3 months after you have been consistently working out. It is also helpful to direct your focus toward building functional strength, flexibility and aerobic

fitness, rather than your body's appearance. Stay focus and be dedicated, and you will witness your physique gradually shrink before your eye!

CHAPTER 3

YOU ARE WHAT YOU EAT

A sensible and health diet makes up the other half of the weight loss equation. In fact, nutrition accounts for a full 60-70% of your physical fitness level. As the old adage goes, you are what you eat. Furthermore, it is not just what you eat; how much and how often you eat also affects how quickly the food is metabolized into energy by the body. So, it is time to take a critical look at your eating habit, look at what is killing you slowly, and do a diet overhaul.

Much like exercising, eating healthy in your 50s must take into account the specific needs of your age, lifestyle and present overall health. Formulating a diet pan is tricky and there really are no one-size-fit all templates for the perfect diet. The best diet plans are the ones which are tailored specifically for the individual, often requiring a thorough health and lifestyle assessment, perhaps some trial-and-error to figure out what's best. In order to overhaul your eating habits though, you need to be armed with the right knowledge on nutrition and proper eating habits to benefit your metabolism.

Listed here are the Dos and Don'ts of healthy eating to make the process as non-complicating as possible. Go through them, assess your current dietary habits, and fine tune them accordingly.

- **Skipping breakfast is bad for you.** When you skip the first meal of the day – after your stomach has been empty for hours – your body goes into energy conservations mode. In other words, your metabolism gets off to a slow start. If you habitually skip breakfast, switch to eating a light breakfast before or shortly after your cardio exercise (as explained in Chapter 2).

- **Space your meals evenly.** Eating large, infrequent meals with big gaps between on meal and the next may cause metabolic slow down. Out body has a built-in survival mechanism that stores calories, so when you starve yourself, survival mode kicks in. No to mention, you may feel stomach discomfort and heartburn from the flatulence. To remedy this, eat smaller and more frequent meals – 4 to 6 servings a day – with no more than 4 hours in between meals. Calories can be converted more quickly to energy this way.

- **Balance is key.** A balance diet is once which supplies your body with protein, carbohydrates, fats and all the necessary vitamins and minerals. According to Harvard University's healthy eating plate dietary plan recommendation, the proper nutritious meal should consists of one-half fruits and non-starchy vegetables, one-quarter of low-fat protein sources and one-quarter of whole grains, brown rice and other complex carbohydrates. That's a great rule of thumb to adhere by when planning your meals.

- **If it does not come from nature, it does not belong on your plate.** Processed foods, refined carbohydrates, and anything filled artificial flavoring, additives and preservatives need to be minimized from your diet. These are stuff that comes in packages, cans and boxes that has a long shelf life, such as instant noodles, microwave dinner, canned soups etc. They only contribute to the formation of diseases in the long-run. It

27

may not be realistic to totally eliminate them from your diet in our modern life today, but at least cut them out by 90% from your overall diet by opting for a natural substitute whenever feasible. For example, you can always buy raw meat to make curry rather than the canned variety. Want pineapples for your fruit salad? Buy whole pineapple and cut it up instead of canned fruits.

- **Eat your age.** It is often advisable to dress appropriately for your age, but few people will tell you to eat appropriately for your age. If you continue to eat like in your 20s and 30s, without increasing your amount of exercise, you will definitely gain weight. As you get older and your metabolism slows, you actually need fewer calories. Long gone are the days when you can binge eat without little to no effect on your waistline. If you just watch your portion size and replace all those pizzas, cheeseburgers and junk foods with loads of fruits, vegetables, and lean proteins, your caloric consumption would already have decreased.

- **No need to count every calorie, just use portion control.** Unless you have severe weight issues and are advised by a qualified dietician, it is not advisable to obsess over the amount of calories consumed. Doing so takes away your enjoyment of food, which in turn can be discouraging to your weight loss attempts. Just be mindful of your portion and lifestyle caloric needs. For instance, if you are only exercising likely, your job and daily activities are not very physical, you need to eat less. As you progress in your exercise program, you may need to eat a little bit more.

- **Watch what you snack on.** Snacking between meals is good for staving off hunger. However, your choice of snack could be contributing to weight gain. Substitute potato chips, candies and chocolate for healthy alternatives, such as rice crackers, fruits, nuts and dark chocolate.

- **Get enough calcium and plenty of protein.** You need calcium to keep bones strong, while protein is needed to facilitate overall bodily functions, including building bones, muscles, skin and blood, and helps regulate a healthy body weight. Foods rich in protein and calcium include fish, eggs, poultry lean meat, mushrooms, cheese, yoghurt and milk.

- **Cook your meals.** Making your own meals gives you full control of what goes into them than when you eat out. There is nothing wrong with dining out, but be careful of the places you dine in. However, you don't really know what goes into your food when you eat at a restaurant. For the duration which you are trying to reach your weight loss goals though, it would be best to minimize eating out and focus on reforming your dietary habits. You will find that as you learn more about nutrition and cut out the bad stuff from your home cooking, you will become more wary and selective of the eateries you go to.

- **Less salt, sugar and flour.** Known as the 'Three Deadly White Food Products', these ingredients are best limited from your food for maximum health impact, regardless of your age. Refined sugar has an addictive effect akin to alcohol and drugs, and high consumption of it is linked to many illnesses. A diet high in salt can increase the risk of high blood pressure, while white flour is absolutely unnecessary to your diet as it has almost no nutritional value.

- **Take your antioxidants.** As we aged, our body is slowly ravaged by free radicals that cause cellular damage to vital organs. Natural antioxidants can neutralize the harmful effects of free radicals. Raw foods, fruits and vegetables are great sources of antioxidant. To get the most antioxidants in your diet, vary the range of colors of raw foods on your plate.

- **Soluble fiber is good for you.** At least 70% of all disease starts from a poor digestive system. Soluble fiber – found mostly in whole grains, fruits and vegetables, oats and berries, beans, nuts, and vegetables like cucumbers and lentils – improves your body's ability to efficiently digest and process foods properly. A good digestive track flushes harmful toxins and chemicals from your body and also helps regulate your body weight.

- **Don't easily trust anything that is "natural".** It is common to see labels on canned foods and bottled juices that claimed to be "natural". If a food item at the supermarket is labeled "natural", that means it is a healthy product, right? No quite so. The Federal Drug Administration (FDA) in the United States has no straight definition for the word 'natural'. So, anything can be labeled as such on the package, whether it is healthy, processed, and really natural or not. Thread carefully and do your homework before buying a food product with those claims. Even better, stick to the kind that was obtained from the wilderness. For example, given a choice between a box of "Natural Fresh Orange Juice" and some oranges you can squeeze for juice, go for the latter.

- **Stay hydrated.** The daily recommended amount of water by most physicians is 8 cups. However, you should increase the amount of water you drink on hot and humid days, and after an intense physical activity. Carbonated and caffeinated beverages will only leave dehydrated as these drinks are diuretic – they draw water out of your body. Dehydration can lead to migraines, low energy and other harmful side effects. So, as a general rule, you should drink 2 cups of water for every cup of coffee, tea or soda.

Weight Loss Pitfalls to Avoid

Just like there are all sorts of fitness fads throughout history, there are a lot of dieting fads which not only jeopardize your weight loss efforts, some of them could even be dangerous. We live in a judgmental world where there is always a pressure to look a certain way, regardless of your age. It is understandable that people tend to fall for a fad diet in a desperate attempt to shed the weight as fast as possible. Sometimes, a dieting fad caught on because some celebrities are following it. You may even received advice from well-meaning, but misinformed friends and family trying to help you achieve your weight loss goals. If you have been recommended a diet plan that some people claimed to live by and think about trying out for yourself, check to make sure it does not advocate any of the following. If it does, do NOT do it; you will only end up disappointed.

- **'Cleansing' diet plans.** Perhaps the most dangerous of all fad diets, cleansing-based eating plans are that that claims to "cleanse" or "detoxifies" your body of gunk that has been stored up for so long, causing you to be a few kilos heavier. These plans usually involve recipes or buying specific products that, when taken, will cause a lot of bowel movement. There is almost no concrete medical-based evidence to support 'cleansing' your body.

- In truth, detoxification happens naturally when the digestive system is functioning optimally, and this can be achieved by staying properly hydrated and eating adequate amounts of soluble fibrous foods. The danger of these diets is that you could be abusing your digestive system by making it work on overdrive, and flushing out the good bacteria in your stomach that is needed to aid digestion. This can cause problems like irritable bowel syndrome or a sluggish digestion in the long-run. If you do lose weight at all using this method, it is only temporary loss of water weight. But by going into the toilet too often, you also run the risk of expelling more water from your body than it is safe, leading to dehydration.

- **Quick-fix supplements.** Whether it is fat-burning pills, detox drinks, meal replacement drinks or slimming shakes, any supplement that claims to make you shed weight in record time should be avoided. The results you get from these supplements usually come with a cost. You may end up suffering all sorts of side effects. Many of these products have no medical backing and work to help you shed a few weight temporarily. If you are on medication, they may interact with the drug you are taking.

- **Eating plans that center on one food item.** This is the sort of diets that advocated eating only open or a few types of foods, such as the banana diet, fruits only meal plan, smoothie cleanse plan or liquid diet. Eating only one type of food to lose weight is not a balanced approach that nourishes your body with all the essential nutrients it needs. You may lose weight quickly with these diets, but you will experience a rebound just as fast. This is because such diet leave you feeling low in energy, making you feel the urge to binge eat.

- **Low fat diets.** It is only logical that to lose weight, you have to cut down on eating fatty foods. However, that could not have been more further from the truth. Fat has an important function to help other nutrients perform their duties and maintain certain bodily functions. Without fat, your immune system will weaken. There is also a link between low fat diet and various health conditions like depression, cancer, drop in good cholesterol, and risk of heart disease. Furthermore, many packaged low fat foods that claim to not contribute to weight gain are actually loaded with additives and large amount of salt (sodium).

- The solution is not to cut fat out, but eat more good fats that will help you lose (bad) fat, build muscle, and recover faster from your workouts. In addition, they are good for your heart and brain health. Good fats are found in fish, nuts, olive oil, peanut butter, flaxseed, avocados, almonds and coconut oil.

- **Calorie-restricting and deprivation eating plans.** Also known as crash dieting, these are eating plans that require you to eat below 1000 calories or restrict yourself to a couple of small meals every day. It goes without saying that depriving your body of the essential nutrients and calories from food means depriving yourself of the energy you need to function normally. Strive to lower your caloric intake to what is necessary, not cutting out a large chunk of your energy needs.

CHAPTER 4

WEIGHT LOSS SABOTEURS

Now that you have learned the two key components to cranking up your metabolism and losing weight, you need to also be aware of other factors that could be compromising your weight loss. Be aware of the six weight loss saboteurs in your lifestyle and work on eliminating them as soon as you can.

Stress

Above all the destructive aspects of life, nothing can top stress. It is the root cause of all illnesses, from hypertension to cancer to mental health disorders. In terms of weight management, stress increases level of a hormone called cortisol in the body. Cortisol is responsible for the storage of extra fat, especially around the belly.

Learning how to manage and combat stress is crucial to your overall health. The best solution is to stick with your workout plan, since exercising is known to increase levels of hormones like dopamine that elevates mood. It is also helpful to adopt mindful practices like meditation. You also want to check yourself to make sure you do not turn to eating or snacking to relieve stress.

Smoking

Nicotine in cigarettes increases the metabolism, albeit in an unhealthy way as it can lead to greater health complications that outweighs the weight loss. Quitting smoking will temporarily lower your metabolism, but that can be easily offset by increasing your daily cardio exercises. After all, when you stop smoking, you will experience increased energy levels that allow you to cope with more intense workout and lose weight the healthy way.

Alcohol Consumption

Beer belly is not just an expression! First of all, alcohol is empty calories – meaning calories with no nutritional value to the body. Secondly, excessive alcohol consumption put a great burden on the liver, which is involved in helping the body burn fat. If you have too much booze in your system, the liver will be kept busy flushing it out first, resulting in more fat being stored in the body. Moreover, at age 50, your liver is not as strong as it was in your college days.

Lack of sleep

Contrary to popular belief, you do not need less sleep as you age. The average adult will need 7-8 hours of uninterrupted quality sleep each night for the body and mind to recuperate. Sleep deprivation increases cortisol levels, increases hunger level, makes the digestive system and consequently the metabolism more sluggish.

To make sure you catch enough Zs, maintain a constant sleep schedule and a comfortable sleep environment, free from the distractions of light-emitting electronics devices. So, no laptops, radio and TV in the room! And talk to your doctor about it if you are having trouble sleeping.

Hormonal Imbalance

We experience a decline in progesterone, testosterone, and other hormones as we age, which sets the body up for storing instead of losing weight. It is important to get your thyroid, adrenal glands, and other hormone levels checked. If you are having trouble losing weight after following a consistent program for a reasonable duration (8-12 weeks) or are shedding pounds at an alarming rate, see a doctor about it. You could be suffering from hormonal imbalance caused by an underlying health condition that you don't know of.

Prescription medication

Some medications, such as antidepressants, beta blockers and steroids, can have the side effect of slowing down the metabolism. However, prescription medications have an important function in your overall health, so don't stop using them without consulting a doctor. Discuss your concerns about the drug's effects on your weight with your doctor, and ask for suggestions to adjust or change your prescription to help improve your metabolism.

CONCLUSION

Trying to lose weight at 50 by overhauling your lifestyle is no easy feat. However, as it is clearly explained in this guide, it is not impossible. Maintaining an ideal weight as you progress into your golden years is not really about turning back the hands of time – nothing can accomplish that. It is more to do with being the best you can be health wise, for the sake of your quality of life and the happiness of your loved ones.

Wouldn't you like to have the energy to travel the world after retirement? To enjoy all that life has to offer rather than be bedridden in hospital? To have the energy and mobility to pursue the activities you enjoy? By taking proper care of yourself through healthy eating and staying active, you can! Stop taking your body for granted and start blasting the fat. There is nothing to stop you but yourself.

www.ingramcontent.com/pod-product-compliance
Lightning Source LLC
Chambersburg PA
CBHW060443290526
45793CB00002B/560